D0644905

HOW TO SURVIVE WITHIN OUR HEALTHCARE SYSTEM

Philip A Scheinberg M.D., F.A.C.S.
Linda A Scheinberg R.N.

ISBN: 1480118958
ISBN-13: 9781480118959
Library of Congress Control Number: 2012919663
CreateSpace Independent Publishing Platform
North Charleston, SC

Reading this booklet may save your life, or the life of someone close to you. Make no mistake the healthcare system in the United States could easily be the very best in the industrialized world. Where we excel is in knowledge, technology and capacity. However, where we seem to be failing is in the mechanism of delivery. The bottom line is that too many people are injured or die within a well-meaning system that recognizes and understands its own problems, but cannot seem to remedy them. The overwhelming majority of people using our system of healthcare simply do not understand how the care is being delivered, where the greatest risks lie, and how to avoid or reduce these risks. Patients often remain uncertain about what questions to ask. As a consumer, you have a lot of "skin" in this game. Your life or the life of a loved one may depend on your willingness to be proactive, to advocate for yourself, and to ask questions. For many of us, healthcare costs are only exceeded by the cost of housing, yet we know little or nothing about what we are so heavily invested in. Somehow we are depending on an over-burdened system to guide us through the minefield. Most of us know more about our cars, favorite sports teams, or the social network than the very system that will hopefully keep us alive.

Our purpose in writing this book is to help the medical consumer understand what appears to be so complex and intimidating. We have distilled into an easily understood format, some of the things everyone should know about being a healthcare recipient, and how to protect oneself from our system's failings. Much of what we offer are insider's tips and information you may otherwise never know. We must also offer a disclaimer, that is, that within our system for care giving, there are so many potential areas for difficulties we cannot possibly cover them all. We can, however, encourage you to be an informed consumer. This means ask questions, pay attention to what is happening, and advocate. You cannot expect your doctor or the system to be watching your back all the time!

We, your authors, share a combined fifty seven year experience in health care delivery. Although we have not seen "everything," we have vast experience and much cumulative wisdom. We have both also chosen to retire from medicine because of persistently growing dissatisfaction with our careers. It is entirely possible your doctor wishes to do the same.

This book is broken down into several very short and concise chapters. The hour or two it will take to read this may make this the most important read of your life.

Respectfully
Philip A Scheinberg, MD, FACS
Linda A Scheinberg, RN

ACKNOWLEDGEMENTS

We would like to express our gratitude to the system of American medicine, the very best the world has to offer. We are both grateful for the superb training we received in our respective areas of medicine and health care provision, and for the incredible privilege granted to us in caring for so many wonderful people over the years. We did not assume this responsibility lightly. We would also like to thank Linda and Steve Larson for their assistance in preparing this manuscript for publication.

TABLE OF CONTENTS

ALARMING STATISTICS

According to the Institute of Medicine (IOM), as many as 100,000 people die each year because of preventable medical incidents. This includes health care acquired infections.

About 1.4 million patient safety incidents reported occurred among 37 million Medicare hospitalizations between the years 2000-2002. An alarming percentage of these patients died.

In one study, patient safety incidents accounted for $8.54 billion in excess in-patient costs to the Medicare system over the three years studied. Extrapolated to the entire US, an extra 19 billion dollars were spent, and more than 575,000 preventable deaths occurred from 2000-2002.

There has been little evidence of improved patient safety since this study.

Medical liability cost the US healthcare system $126 billion in 2002.

A very high percentage of Orthopedic Surgeons avoid caring for high-risk patients for fear of liability repercussions. (American Academy of Orthopedic Surgeons)

If these alarming statistics applied to automobile or air travel, we would all be engaged in a better understanding of the problems involved. We would at least have the option to stay home or to walk to our destination. As consumers however, we seem to blindly believe that all is fine within our system of healthcare and we shall always be in good and safe hands. This is just not always true.

"Providers" (we used to refer to them as "doctors and nurses") in many instances are overworked, frustrated, and economically disincentivized. This means undercompensated and unappreciated.

A recent survey published in the June, 2012 Bulletin of The American College of Surgeons reveals that 9 out of 10 survey responders indicate an unwillingness to recommend health care as a profession. In addition, 43% of responders indicate that they are contemplating retiring within the next five years as a result of transformative changes occurring within the US health care system.

Some providers are inadequately trained, poorly skilled, or impaired in some way.

The medical consumer is often uneducated about the healthcare system, and unrepresented by any meaningful advocacy system.

The legal tort system is often self-serving and has brought no meaningful positive change to health care quality or availability. To the contrary, this legal system has participated in making many medical services even more difficult to receive.

The insurance industry is poorly understood by the consumer and often fails to facilitate or improve care access. Poor reimbursement for many services, make these services difficult to obtain. Health insurance has become so costly, that it now represents a major monthly household cost for those who can afford it.

THE AUTHORS

Philip A Scheinberg, MD, FACS grew up in Miami Florida, the son of a physician. I knew early on that the practice of medicine was for me. My father, being a highly esteemed medical academician, obviously loved what he did and surrounded himself with other accomplished doctors. Medicine was a highly respected career and I was proud of him. In many ways I wanted to be like him. After high school, I became a pre-med student at Emory University in Atlanta, Georgia, and upon completion of my studies, was fortunate enough to be accepted into the freshman class at The University of Miami School of Medicine in 1970. Having always enjoyed working with my hands, I found myself drawn to a career in Surgery. After completing my Surgical Internship in Denver Colorado, I began my specialty training as a resident in Otolaryngology, Head and Neck Surgery (Ear, Nose and Throat) at Stanford University in Palo Alto, California. The medical training experience was a grueling one, each year becoming more demanding as my skills and responsibilities grew. The training regimen demanded nothing less than excellence and total immersion. There was very little time for self or family, but I, like most others doing the same, got through it with a wonderful education and the necessary skills to help others. In 1979 I successfully took my specialty board examination and became a proud Fellow of the American Academy of Otolaryngology. I was 32 years old and finally ready to begin my independent practice. I was fortunate to practice both in Santa Cruz and Santa Barbara, California until my retirement from active medical practice in 2005. I also enjoyed the distinct privilege of serving on the clinical faculty at Stanford for many years, working with the residents that followed me. From the time I began in medicine in 1970, until my retirement in 2005, I participated in caring for many people, sharing in their lives, and observing many changes in medicine as a whole. My wonderful wife, Linda, is a Registered Nurse with many years of experience in the acute care hospital setting, as well as in the clinic with me. She too has had a vast clinical experience in medicine at many levels and has a perspective that most physicians simply do not have.

So, why would I have retired so early, with potentially many productive years in medicine left ahead of me? The bottom line: I simply was no longer enjoying what I was doing professionally, and after experiencing a serious illness myself, I decided it was now time to do something else with my life. Medicine had been socially evolving into something that grew more distasteful to me each passing year. In my eyes, physician autonomy, prestige and professional satisfaction were being eroded by many external forces. Some of these were political, many economic, and some social. I, like many physicians, cherished my independence as a doctor, my abilities to guide my patients through profound challenges of their own, and to indulge in the professional relationships and satisfaction that this wonderful career in medicine had allowed me to enjoy. As politics and the insurance industry became more intrusive in the way I practiced my craft as a surgeon, I found myself growing more professionally impotent and dissatisfied. Sadly, I believe these feelings are now very pervasive throughout the practice of medicine at almost every level. Although many of my wonderful colleagues soldier on with their medical careers, I sense that the professional joy and satisfaction once so pervasive in medicine has now reached a very low ebb indeed. Combining this factor with many other demands, placed on a very finite resource, has created a volatile and potentially dangerous environment in which we seek our health care. To this end, Linda and I have written this short manual to assist you. Read it for what it is. It does not attempt to address every potential pitfall a health care consumer may encounter, but more to act as a simple and perhaps folksy survival manual as the health care environment grows ever darker. A last disclaimer: Again this is intended to make you aware of potential medical issues. In fact, medical practice models and styles can vary throughout the US. The streets may be "meaner" in some areas than in others. But, being more informed is always a good thing.

Both of us feel very qualified in sharing with you our insights and recommendations. In so many ways we feel that this short book will allow us to continue with our abilities to improve, if not preserve life, maybe even yours.

BEFORE WE BEGIN, A FEW BASICS

What can I do as an informed consumer? All of the basics apply here. Understand the mechanisms of care access as outlined by your insurance plan, if you have one. What are your responsibilities relative to the plan? If you don't know, or it is not clear to you from reading the information provided to you by your insurance company, ask! Call your insurance company or broker, or find out from Human Resources at work. If you have insurance, there are rules to follow and there is written information available. This means that you will actually have to read and understand your insurance manual. Although this sounds daunting, it remains your responsibility to understand the important components of your plan. I cannot emphasize enough how important this is. Time spent doing this will prevent potentially serious misunderstandings later on.

If you are a Medicare beneficiary, understand how Medicare works. It is not very complicated, but there are pitfalls to avoid within the system. Read and/or ask.

Know which physicians, hospitals, laboratories and outpatient providers are in your network of caregivers, and who is not. You may not choose to enroll or remain within your current insurance provider network once you understand this. Try to sort this out as early as possible. The doctor or hospital of your choice may not be a contracted provider for the insurance plan you may be considering. If you receive care from a non-contracted provider (out of network), the costs to you as a patient may be substantially higher than care delivered in network by a contracted provider.

Ask questions. Look it up online. Knowing this information may save you lots of money and it may save your life. You just need to sit down and do it. Someone in the family must understand how the system works. Eventually it will be necessary, guaranteed.

YOUR DOCTOR

As a physician, I feel well qualified to share some very useful insights here. Although there are many wonderful aspects to the practice of medicine, we as physicians have been confronted with a growing series of professional challenges which impact on physician autonomy, professional satisfaction, care access and methodology of health care delivery. Let's begin with an analogy which will help you to better understand part of the medical marketplace. We will refer back to this analogy a bit later in the text. It is 10:00 pm, and your kitchen sink drain has backed up creating a mess. You pick up your phone and call your plumber, who surprisingly answers the phone, and you say to him, "I am having trouble with my sink and you must come repair it right now. If my homeowner's policy pays me for this, I will pay a small portion of your bill. Also, if you are not here in the next 30 minutes, or if I am not happy with your work, I will sue you." One can only imagine the plumber's response to this call.

The vast majority of physicians, being either MDs (Doctors of Medicine) or DOs (Doctors of Osteopathy) are well-trained, well-meaning and caring individuals. A career in medicine begins with an altruistic journey involving grueling study and training, self-deprivation and personal sacrifice. The US offers the finest and most comprehensive medical training in the world, period. You can be certain that a US board-certified physician will be well trained. That however does not guarantee that he or she will be completely attentive or responsive to your needs as a patient. If your doctor in fact is attentive, that is terrific. If he or she is not, there may be a number of reasons accounting for this.

Physicians today face an ever growing number of professional challenges. Demands placed on their time can often become virtually overwhelming. Physicians, being people like anyone else, can be influenced by economic, social, family, and professional demands. I think it may be fair to say, that in many situations, physicians can be overworked and underpaid. Let's face it, we all have bills to pay, and demands to meet. Although no doctor begins his or her career expecting to be influenced by these eventualities, they sadly have become a fact of life.

When very significant demands are placed on an individual, with constant pressure being applied to work incentives (read payment for services), the willingness to continually extend oneself to be responsive and available 24/7 can be compromised. Surely you understand that as well as I. Few people appreciate working within a system where there is little recognition for extraordinary efforts and an overwhelming sense of looming legal penalty. Until Congress, our insurance, and legal "industries" reevaluate some of these issues, there will remain difficulties with the full scope of quality medical care access and delivery.

At this point I would like to refer back to the plumber analogy. Please go back and reread it. This time the upset homeowner is you the patient and the plumber has now become your doctor. This is a very appropriate analogy. Not all doctors may see it this way, but I can assure you, many do. Therein lies a problem. Something has happened to the sacred physician-patient relationship. With the long-standing economic and political intrusion of the powerful insurance industry between the doctor and the patient, now further complicated by governmental manipulation of our "sacred trust," the chasm is growing wider. More about this later.

With all that being said, what can you as the patient do to improve your odds of a quality care outcome? What can the patient do to get the most from his relationship with his or her physician? There is much you can do to further tip the odds in your favor.

WHO IS YOUR PHYSICIAN?

Knowing that your doctor is an MD or a DO, and little else about him or her, is just plain insufficient, if not stupid. Medicine, like every other highly technical enterprise, has tremendously evolved over the last generation. No longer can the kindly family "Doc" be expected to know all he needs to know. We live in the age of specialization where our knowledge has become so vast, that many specialists now focus on subspecialties within their specialty. Access to specialists is far easier in more urban environments than rural ones. Depending on where we choose to live, we access what we can. The key is in knowing what questions to ask. As a physician, when I as a patient, meet a new doctor who will care for me, I would like to know the following;

1. Where was this doctor trained?
2. What are his medical board qualifications?
3. How long has he been in practice?
4. Which hospitals or medical centers does he affiliate with?
5. What are his office policies regarding insurance contracts and payment for services?
6. How may I reach him both during and after office hours, and with whom does he share his on call coverage?

This information should be easily available from the physician or his office staff. Being the inquisitive fellow that I am, I may also check online through the State Medical Board or local Medical Society about this doctor's reputation. Has there been a history of adverse litigation against him? This information is not always easy to get, but if you are interested, there are ways of finding out. Ask around your community. You would likely not entrust your new BMW to the shade tree mechanic down the street, unless you knew he was properly trained.

7. You will also want to know who will care for you if you are admitted to the hospital. Will it be the doctor you know or will it be a Hospitalist? The Hospitalist is usually an Internist or specialty Internist who is skilled at caring for both in-patients (patients in the hospital), and very sick patients. This doctor may not be your regular physician, as many hospitals now use a Hospitalist program for care consistency, improved outcomes, and cost containment. This is a newer concept in in-patient care delivery, and is rapidly becoming a standard of care.
8. You must also know who your doctor cross covers with when your doctor is not available. I would like to know as much as possible about this doctor or group of doctors as well. Makes sense doesn't it?

9. Is my doctor a solo practitioner or in a group practice?
10. What are his or her insurance contracted affiliations and does he accept my plan? This information is available to you in your insurance plan provider manual. Basically, this booklet will tell you with whom your plan contracts for service, (in network), and unless otherwise specified, everyone else is out of network. You must be aware of this prior to going to the doctor, otherwise you may not be able to see that doctor, or it may result in unexpected costs to you. Most medical office staff will ask what insurance plan you have prior to scheduling an appointment. This does not always mean, however, that this doctor accepts your insurance, so ask. Understand your insurance plan. This is your responsibility, not your doctor's. Insurance plans can be complex, so do your homework.

Speaking about insurance plans; understand if your doctor is part of a PPO (Preferred Provider Organization) or an HMO (Health Maintenance Organization). There is a very big difference between these two basic entities and how you will receive your care. We will talk more about them later in the chapter on Insurance.

Lastly, I cannot stress this point enough. Your primary care doctor cannot be expected to have vast and comprehensive expertise in all aspects of medicine. There is just too much to know. If you as the patient have a history, or perhaps strong family history of an illness that historically would be managed by a specialist, then ask, demand if necessary, to see the appropriate specialist for your screening evaluation. For example; prostate cancer is a common and potentially lethal disease in men, which when identified and treated early can be completely curable. With all due respect, most primary care physicians do not possess the clinical expertise to identify this disease early on with a digital rectal examination. This examination and evaluation is best left to the Urologist.......period. If you have a family history of breast cancer, the best diagnostician will be the Gynecologist or Surgeon. Not being proactive here, for yourself or loved one, MAY COST A LIFE! There is no room for sensitive egos. Ask for what you want. Your primary care doctor will be happy to comply and assist you. If he or she is not, find another doctor.

Always be prepared for your medical appointments. Be prepared to ask appropriate questions. Bring pen and paper with you and write things down if need be, so you get the most from your visit. Recognize also that your doctor will generally have a specified amount of time to spend with you. Use this time wisely. You have a big stake in your or your loved one's medical problem. Don't expect your doctor to shoulder it alone for you. Participate, be there, ask questions and become informed.

WHAT KIND OF DOCTOR IS YOUR DOCTOR?

The majority of physicians in the U.S. are MDs, Doctors of Medicine. To be a legally practicing physician, an MD must be appropriately trained and licensed within the state or states in which they practice medicine. Licensure requires graduation from an approved medical school and a certain amount of post-graduate training depending on the specialty. In most instances this consists of a year of internship and usually two or more years of specialty residency training in a teaching hospital. Many physicians extend their specialty training even further with a year or more of fellowship training. By the time this lengthy training process is completed, the physician is usually in his mid-thirties and well-trained within his chosen specialty. Likely as well, the physician will have completed the necessary specialty board examination allowing that physician to be a member of his or her specialty College or Society.

This specialty board certification is generally the patient's assurance that this doctor has completed the rigorous training necessary to practice his respective craft with the expected level of skill, judgment and knowledge. After completion of the specialty board certification, and after a year or more of medical specialty practice, the physician can also choose to become a Fellow of the American College of Surgeons, (FACS), or College of Physicians, (FACP). These initials after MD are even further acknowledgement of your doctor's prestige, skill and training. These college affiliations are not earned by all Surgeons or Physicians.

In light of the vast amount of medical knowledge that exists, most physicians choose to be specialists. Many choose specialties within specialties and have finely honed their respective levels of skill and knowledge. When you are confronted with an illness or problem, generally there exists a specialty doctor within your community. If not, one may be found at a regional Medical Center.

Your family doctor may be an FP, Family Practitioner, or a GP, General Practitioner, and skilled at well-patient care, preventative medicine and many other areas commonplace in general practice. Many years ago, it was the GP who provided much of a patient's care before the emergence of medical specialties. Now, required specialty care is generally referred to the appropriate specialist.

Your physician may be an Internist with specialty training focused in a branch of Internal Medicine. Internists have often had additional training beyond that of the Family or General Practitioner. Subspecialties within Internal Medicine may include; Cardiology, Gastroenterology, Endocrinology, Pediatrics, Oncology, Rheumatology, Hematology, Pulmonology,

Critical Care Medicine, Dermatology, Nephrology, Neurology, Geriatrics, etc.

Likely, if you find yourself hospitalized as a patient, the doctor overseeing your care may be a hospital- based physician called a Hospitalist. Hospitalists may be more efficient at caring for sick people in the hospital environment than the community-based Internist. Your Internist or Family Physician will be consulting with the Hospitalist, and providing additional needed information about you and your illness.

Most surgeons see patients on a referral basis for problems within their area of specialty and do not provide primary care. The OB/Gyn is a surgeon who offers some component of primary care for female patients. Obviously, this is the doctor to see for Obstetrical and Gynecologic needs and preventative care in this area. Other examples of surgical specialties are: Orthopedics, Otolaryngology (Ear Nose and Throat), General Surgery, Cardio-Thoracic Surgery, Urology, Plastic and Reconstructive Surgery, Neurosurgery, etc. Most trauma specialists are Surgeons. The list goes on.

Lastly, there exists a group of generally hospital-based doctors such as Radiologists, Anesthesiologists, Pathologists and the previously mentioned Hospitalist. Emergency room physicians fall into this category as well, and one of these may be the first doctor who cares for you in a critical care situation.

In many instances, particularly in large clinic or managed care practices, the patient may receive an evaluation or care from a physician extender, specifically a Nurse Practitioner (NP) or a Physician's Assistant (PA). These well-trained providers are generally skilled in basic patient encounters such as routine history and physical exams, screening evaluations, wound and peri-operative care to mention a few. Again, encounters with physician extenders are going to be more commonplace in high-volume patient practices and managed care situations. Although not doctors, they are usually quite skillful at what they do. There is a big difference in their training as compared to a physicians' however. Know who is caring for you. Ultimately a doctor will oversee the Physician Extender's care and decision making in most instances. The PA and NP can greatly extend the reach of medical services in many instances, and often provide for those who may otherwise go without any care.

Is there a difference in physician training? Absolutely. Although there are many excellent foreign medical graduates practicing medicine in the US, American medical training is generally unsurpassed anywhere in the world today. Be certain that if you are seeing a medical specialist, he or she is appropriately trained and board certified by the respective specialty board. This assures that you are receiving the most skillful care. If you do not know what your doctor's qualifications are, ask! Not doing so could leave you with serious regrets. Board certification is your "Good Housekeeping" seal of approval.

How do I get to see the doctor of my choice? This may or may not be possible, depending on your health insurance plan, the physician's availability, whether he or she is accepting new patients, and in certain instances, whether or not you and your physician get along with one another. Physicians can still reserve the right to accept and treat anyone they so choose, or choose not to treat. Many insurance plans offer such poor levels of contractual physician reimbursement, that some doctors may choose not to provide for patients with these plans.

Medicare is beginning to fall into this category as well. Physicians, as of now at least, are not legally mandated to come to the office every day and treat everyone who wants to be seen. Doctors still have some choice in the matter, just as does the patient.

If a physician is providing active and ongoing care to a patient, and for whatever reason, there exists a conflict between the physician and the patient, the physician must either continue to provide care continuity until the illness is resolved, or arrange care coverage for that patient with another doctor. Your doctor cannot legally or ethically abandon you in the midst of the acute care process. Mutual respect and communication will help establish comfortable care relationships with your doctors. Like anyone else, physicians are people and do not respond well to disrespectful, threatening, or demanding behavior from their patients. Conflicted situations may result in appropriate and legal termination of the doctor/patient relationship. Patients who make litigious threats or display inappropriate or otherwise threatening behavior, may find themselves looking for another doctor. This of course is a two way street. If you feel you are not receiving the quality care you deserve, you should bring it to the attention of the physician or staff or find another doctor if the need arises.

Lastly, there is the issue of "time". Your doctor may or may not always be on time or on schedule to see you. Delivering health care does not always keep to a precise time frame. Likely your doctor is doing the best he can to be mindful of your time as well. As a patient, if you are on a tight schedule, call your doctor ahead of your appointment and check to be certain the doctor will see you at the appointed time. Be on time for your appointments, have with you your needed medical records, and be engaged with the physician or caregiver in resolving your problem. Be courteous to the office staff as they should be to you. As is human nature, physicians and staff respond best to the patients they like.

So, how do you get to see the doctor of your choice? Your insurance plan will provide a list of contracted providers for you to choose from. If the doctor of your choice is not listed as a provider, you should call his or her office and ask if the doctor will see you and accept your insurance payment. The doctor may not accept your insurance as payment in full, and request that you pay the non-covered difference. Whether your doctor is independent, in a group, or in a clinic, insurance provider contracts generally limit who can be seen as patients. Please keep in mind, that if your physician of choice is not contracted with your insurance carrier, he is under no obligation to accept your insurance as payment for service.

If the doctor is a Medicare provider, and at this writing most are, he or she must accept Medicare payment as payment in full, less the 20% patient co-pay that the patient must pay. With persistent reductions in payment by Medicare, there will be fewer doctors willing to care for Medicare patients. Those that do provide for Medicare patients may not always be willing to spend the time necessary to deliver the personalized care we have all come to expect. The medical consumer must be careful that this is not the case. Self- advocacy, or family support and advocacy can play a very important role in maximizing a quality care outcome. More on the issues of advocacy will be discussed in the final chapter.

Patients dependent on state-funded Medicaid will have fewer options yet, as payment for services is so low. Most Medicaid beneficiaries will receive their care through facilities specifically designed to provide for these patients. Specialty care will often be provided by outside physicians who are willing to see Medicaid patients.

Nurses and the Team

The importance of the role of the Registered Nurse cannot be overstated. Whether working in the hospital setting or in an outpatient capacity, RNs are generally the lead caregivers. They work with Licensed Vocational Nurses (LVNs) and Certified Nursing Assistants (CNAs) and other staff members who are all important team participants. Highly trained and skillful RNs are able to observe and assess the condition and needs of their patients; communicate with Physicians; make suggestions where appropriate; implement Doctors' orders and individually designed components of the specific care plan for the patient. The role of the nurse includes all aspects of patient care, from comfort measures to often complicated monitor reading and calibration, medication and IV fluid and blood product administration, complex treatments and wound care, emotional support and grief counseling, and education of patients and family members and student nurses. The RN can stand between a patient and a poor outcome. The RN will likely be the first responder in an emergency. In some instances, the RN must provide resuscitation measures and make other critical care decisions to save a person's life. At the same time the nurse is required to keep records of all that occurs on that particular shift. Currently hospital records are mostly electronic, which requires additional input from the nursing staff. This new technological demand clearly cuts into the time nurses have to spend with their patients, and may diminish the personal nature of the care received. This brief overview touches only on the basics. Tasked with so many responsibilities, it is no wonder that caregivers cannot always provide patients with everything, such as a much-needed shampoo. This is disappointing to both patient and caregiver.

Currently our country suffers from a growing nursing shortage. This concerning trend often has necessitated the importation of nursing staff called "travelers". These important caregivers may sometimes come from other countries. Language skills and communication can be challenging. Another concerning fact is that nurses tend to be over-worked with their skills stretched thin by unfavorable nurse to patient ratios.

In addition, medication errors comprise some of the most serious care delivery threats to the patient and can result in injury or death. Mistakes occur in part, because the staff is often overburdened and rushing to meet the demands of modern medicine in an environment of cost containment. Hospital- borne infections, spread by well-meaning staff or visitors, are another very serious threat to the hospitalized patient. Caregivers are at risk as well. An example is when a nurse sustains an inadvertently self-inflicted needle stick from a needle that was first used on a patient who carries HIV or Hepatitis C virus. This can place the nurse's health and life in jeopardy.

So, how can patients improve their own care? When allowed, the presence of a family member or advocate in the patient's room can be reassuring and helpful. When possible, family members will want to advocate for their loved ones or specify a designated advocate. It is important that family and staff are mutually respectful, diplomatic and not inappropriately intrusive. It is helpful to remember that the staff is often pushed to deliver care to the next person in need, so understand that time and timing can be an issue.

Family members can become a helpful part of the team, especially when a lengthy stay is involved. If there is an issue that is not being handled in a clear and proper fashion, family advocates can and should ask to speak to the Nursing Supervisor or the Physician in charge of the patient's care.

In short: It really is a team effort. Hospital stays can be complex. Caregivers are tasked with many patients and situations. Nurses are in short supply. Patient advocates can play a crucial role in speaking for those who often are not able to do this for themselves. This all adds up to a more effective effort in helping patients heal and recover.

THE HOSPITAL

The hospital is the health care environment where you, the patient, are at the greatest risk. This is particularly true of the inpatient setting, which is when one has been admitted for hospital specific care. Generally the hospital is a large and very busy place where providers care for numerous people, including you. It is this very feature that places all patients at risk. Some risk is unavoidable, some is not. Risk management requires some effort on the part of the patient, and/or a strong advocacy on the part of the patient's family or friends, particularly when patients are unable to advocate for themselves. When the patient is too sick or incapable of self-advocacy, this is the time when a responsible family member or close friend must be present in the patient's room as much as possible, if not at all times. Even if there is resistance on the part of the hospital personnel, respectfully request that you wish to spend as much time with your loved one as is possible based on hospital protocol and privacy allowances. The patient or advocate should diplomatically express to the caregivers their concerns and awareness regarding the potential risks associated with hospitalization. This communication alone can result in an increase in the diligence in providing quality care.

What kinds of untoward events can occur inadvertently in a hospital environment that a friend or family advocate can help overcome? Let's briefly talk about some of the more common omissions and errors seen in hospital based care giving.

Perhaps the greatest risk to the hospitalized patient is that of hospital acquired infections. This problem has become so prevalent that some statistics show it to be the fourth leading cause of death in America. Hospital borne infections, most commonly MRSA (Methicillin Resistant Staph Aureus) and C. diff. (Clostridium Difficile) have become epidemic in most hospitals around the country and in chronic care environments. We are now seeing additional new infections that are beginning to regularly appear in the hospital environment, some originating in other countries. These preventable bacterial infections can be life-threatening, particularly in surgical patients, those with "central lines" which are indwelling vascular catheters to monitor vascular pressures and administer medications, in patients with urinary catheters, or those whose immune system may be compromised, or in- patients receiving antibiotic treatment for other infections. The longer the patient is in the hospital, the greater the risk. Generally MRSA, C. diff., or other infections can be transmitted from one patient to another by well-meaning care givers, doctors, nurses and nursing assistants etc., who fail to adequately wash their hands between patient contacts. As the patient, or patient advocate, insist that any caregiver that contacts the patient, WASH THEIR HANDS thoroughly with proper antibacterial soap and water before any contact, even if they are putting on gloves for the contact which is the proper standard of care. This is elementary in care giving, but can be overlooked. Prior to a new patient occupying a room, the area should have been thoroughly cleaned and prepared for the new patient. You can add to this process by CAREFULLY WIPING DOWN THE BED RAILS, HEADBOARD, NIGHT STAND, TRAY TABLE, TELEPHONE, TV REMOTE, BATHROOM KNOBS AND FIXTURES WITH ANTISEPTIC WIPES. Come prepared with your own antiseptic wipes. If a care giver appears acutely ill, this should be brought to the attention of the Nursing Supervisor. As the relative shortage of health care providers grows, those available to provide this important work will be pushed to work harder, longer and faster. If you do not believe this is and will become a worsening problem, you are dead wrong!

Medication errors are another unfortunate consequence of the overburdened hospital environment. Often, but not always, certain checks and balances exist in passing medication to sick patients. It is important that the patient advocate present, respectfully and diplomatically have the nurse double check for medication type and dosage prior to administering the drugs, be they oral (by mouth) or injectable. Medication errors are a major source of preventable injuries to patients in the hospital, and can and should be significantly reduced. The advocate should have a piece of paper with the patient's medications listed, including drug allergies and adverse reactions. If the doctor orders new medications while the patient is hospitalized, which is highly likely, be certain to add these meds to your list. Physicians, pharmacists and nurses should be aware of adverse drug reactions, but it is possible that an observant family member may be the first to notice the emergence of adverse symptoms. This will take some effort on the part of the advocate. Wouldn't you want someone doing this for you?

Blood and blood product (plasma, platelets, etc.) transfusions can be life-saving as well as life-threatening. If a surgical procedure is being planned far enough in advance, and blood or blood products are anticipated, speak with your surgeon about autologous blood donation, that is donating blood to yourself in advance, and having it labeled and banked for your future usage. If autologous donation is not a practical consideration, consider a known volunteer donor with your blood type, such as a healthy friend or family member. Although banked blood is screened for Hepatitis C and HIV (AIDS) by screening donors, there unfortunately is no guarantee that the unknown donor blood you receive is not tainted. Fortunately this catastrophe is rare. If the patient has made an autologous pre-need donation, there will have been issued at the time of donation an ID tag attached to the unit of blood. A copy of this ID tag should also have been given to the donor and should be double checked by the patient or advocate at the time the blood is administered. The same can be said for volunteer blood products. Check these tags against the blood being given whenever possible. Although there exists specific protocol for nurses picking up the blood in the lab and hanging the unit at the bedside, another set of eyes and ears cannot hurt.

Here is a solution to another very unfortunate type of error which can occur both in the hospital and out- patient surgical environment. That surprising error is a surgical procedure intended for one limb, or eye, or ear etc., but is inadvertently performed on the wrong side. Many facilities mark the intended surgical site pre operatively, and confirm this with the patient. Sometimes they do not. This very regrettable error can be prevented by being certain that the pre op nurse confirms the intended surgical site in some way before the patient enters the operating room. Always be certain this gets done.

University Medical Centers, e.g. teaching hospitals, function differently from community hospitals. Teaching hospital means exactly that. This is a very sophisticated medical center which trains new physicians and surgeons in their respective areas of interest. Generally patients admitted to a teaching hospital are there because the facility offers unique care and services, sometimes investigational, but usually "cutting edge." Much of the care provided to the patients in these fantastic facilities is from the "house staff," a team of fellows, resident physicians, interns, and medical students. This care is generally overseen by the attending faculty physicians and other experts. These medical centers are usually teaming with activity and can present a bewildering exposure to a vast array of highly sophisticated equipment, clinical experiences and hands on medical care provided by large teams of specialty physicians. In light of the expansive nature of this kind of care, sometimes far from home, the assistance of a cool-headed and well prepared family member or advocate can make the experience less intimidating and more productive for the patient. It is also very important to remember that in light of the exposure to many different care givers and delivery of fast-paced high tech medicine, the attentive advocate is critical to help "protect" the patient and ensure the best possible outcome. This is after all a hospital inpatient experience similar to the one in one's own community. The same risk factors apply, if not more so. Ask questions, be vigilant, observe and advocate.

In addition, a hospital is not a place to bring small children. The risk of a child contracting an infection is not insignificant. Children also can be carrying childhood illnesses which can further compromise the health of hospitalized patients.

HOSPITAL ADMISSION VERSES OBSERVATION

Medicare law has created a conundrum for hospitals, physicians, and Medicare patient beneficiaries. The law mandates that a Medicare patient must be ADMITTED to the hospital by their physician to be eligible for full Medicare Part A benefits. In order for a patient to be eligible to receive ongoing outpatient skilled nursing care, they must have previously been admitted to the hospital for at least three (3) days. To be eligible for post hospitalization Medicare reimbursed drug benefits, the patient must have been admitted to the hospital. Over the last few years hospitals have been categorizing less seriously ill patients as OBSERVATION patients instead of as admitted patients. Although these patients believe they have been admitted to the hospital and are receiving in-patient care, they are in some cases being classified as observation patients, even if they are in the hospital for several days. Hospitals have chosen to utilize this newer observation category instead of traditional admission for a number of reasons, mostly related to Medicare rules and the current Affordable Care Act regulations (Obamacare). Medicare reimburses hospitals under Part A for patients ADMITTED by their physicians. If a patient is held in the hospital under the category of OBSERVATION, the patient may be held responsible for some or all of the charges, and the hospital may receive lower Part A reimbursements. The bottom line is; if you are an observation patient, you will likely be held responsible for some of the costs of the hospitalization, and will not be entitled to Medicare- covered discharge medications or extended care services. There are additional reasons why hospitals have chosen to utilize this very frustrating methodology of handling Medicare patients. There are now very draconian Medicare rules penalizing hospitals and providers for any patient readmitted to the hospital within 30 days of discharge. A patient previously held in the hospital as an observation patient, but now readmitted for the same, or even a different diagnosis, will likely escape a utilization audit from Medicare. Unfortunately, the costs for the patient to be hospitalized for observation may fall entirely on them. It is essential that any Medicare beneficiary who requires hospitalization for an illness be clear on whether they will be ADMITTED by an order from their physician, or held for OBSERVATION. Although the patient may not be aware of any difference in the hospital experience, there potentially will be a huge difference in cost to the patient and their family. This is now a nationwide practice, and is one of the unfortunate consequences of an overburdened system, poor reimbursement levels, and many new regulations. The consumer is caught in the middle here. We can only encourage you to be aware of the admission status and be prepared to strongly advocate for your own interests.

KEEP YOUR OWN MEDICAL RECORDS

Accumulate and keep in an organized fashion all pertinent medical records, current medications, names of physicians who have taken care of you in the past with phone numbers, known drug allergies or intolerances, laboratory tests, pathology reports, X-ray reports (Radiology), etc. This information, kept in a file and brought with you, can make a huge difference in how productive a visit to a new doctor will be. Having this information at your fingertips can save vast amounts of time and energy. If an emergency occurs, necessitating a hospital visit or admission, bringing this critical information can save your life. Although we now live in the age of the electronic medical record, complete data bases are rarely available, particularly in an emergent situation. Everyone should have their own medical file. Your doctor may wish to make copies of information in this file so that your records with him are more complete and accurate. He, in turn, may provide you with hard copy, or e-mailed information as necessary. Do not depend on the completeness or immediate availability of the electronic medical record.

THE SECOND OPINION

Perhaps no other form of self-advocacy is better known than the second opinion. When there appears to be uncertainty about a diagnosis or treatment plan, we know to ask for another medical opinion, usually from a medical expert in the field of concern. That being said, the patient should however request and seek an additional evaluation and opinion whenever there has been made a diagnosis of a life-threatening condition, or a potentially complex procedure has been recommended. There are no hard and fast rules here except this; if you feel another opinion may be warranted, then get it. Be direct with your physician, share your concern, and request guidance in obtaining this additional evaluation and opinion. Perhaps he or she may wish to refer you to a tertiary facility such as a university medical center or a facility focused on your specific diagnosis. Medical science is not always perfect, and it is irrational for anyone to

expect infallibility. But getting another opinion is your preroga-
tive. Use it wisely.

If your physician has referred you to another facility or doctor, be certain you bring with you all pertinent medical records,
X rays, scans and MRI's, pathology reports, and the actual
pathology slides themselves. This will go a long way in facili-
tating your subsequent visit and may eliminate the need for further expensive tests.

Last, when the subsequent opinion is profoundly different
from the first, you must consider a third opinion. This is a judgment call that now must be made by you and your doctor.

CARING FOR OUR ELDERLY

Medical technology in conjunction with the aging "baby boomers" will create a growing challenge to the rapidly changing medical culture. More aptly stated, this challenge may be perceived as a burden. Here is another area where well directed family support and advocacy will be very important to the comfort and well-being of our elderly.

It is common knowledge that a very significant percentage of medical care is consumed in the remaining few years of life. For many elderly patients, they will find themselves without their spouses and living in chronic or long term care facilities or nursing homes. This is big business, and frequently provided in a profit-driven environment, sometimes leaving room for neglect or mismanagement of the care for the elderly patient. We are not indicting all nursing homes or long term care facilities, but it is important to recognize that the infirmed or elderly have special needs and often complex medical and social issues which place them at risk. It is also important to see to it that your loved one is in fact receiving the needed care, love and attention expected, as well as properly dosed medications for acute and chronic conditions such as high blood pressure, heart disease, diabetes, and psychiatric conditions.

Nutritional needs may vary and many older patients may have dietary restrictions, preferences, or special needs. The nutritionist on staff will be very helpful with these decisions. Appealing foods are critical to everyone's well-being.

Good hygiene is necessary for optimal health and comfort. These needs can be complex and time-consuming for some patients, nevertheless, absolutely essential. Family members or advocates must be careful to observe for good hygienic care. Areas of concern to be mindful of are dental and oral care, bowel and bladder management, as well as the basics of regular bathing and the proper sanitation of bedding and clothing. Proper hygiene will go a long way to maintain comfort, dignity and good health, as well as reduce the chances of communicable diseases, skin breakdown and other issues. Individuals who must use indwelling urinary catheters are very much prone to life-threatening urinary tract infections. Proper and carefully supervised catheter care is essential. Catheter management should be prescribed by the physician or care giver, and demonstrated to those who will provide this critical service. There is no room for carelessness here. The same can be said about bed sore prevention and management, as this is an inevitable result of patient neglect and immobility. If you or your loved one have either of these special needs, then absolute vigilance is necessary to prevent an unfortunate outcome. Irregularity is a common problem especially in patients who are in bed or sitting much of the time. Constipation leads to lack of appetite, discomfort and possibly impaction and inability to defecate. Inquire about your loved one, especially if they cannot advocate for themselves.

Social integration and loving family support are essential human needs, just as important as the other areas already mentioned. This includes provisions for mobility and exercise, social programs, entertainment, integration with others, and the exposure to caring staff and access to clergy members where desired.

For those individuals living independently, all of the aforementioned considerations must be thought about. In addition, seeing to it that environmental safety issues are addressed and provisions made to reduce the chance of falls and burns. Falls are one of the greatest dangers we face as we age. With advancing years, our reaction times diminish greatly as do our balance and strength, making us more prone to falls and the injuries they can produce. These injuries often result in severe disabilities and may also bring about a premature death. If family members or friends are unstable on their feet, then it is critical to see to it that either a walker or wheelchair, electric or otherwise is provided for their usage. Most people cling tenaciously to their independence, and will unknowingly jeopardize their own well-being in the process. These devices are all commonly available through pharmacies, durable medical goods suppliers or companies that specialize in home health products. Check with your doctor, home health service, phone book or Internet. Also be sure that the temperature of the water heater in the home is set at a point where the individual of concern cannot inadvertently burn or scald him or herself while bathing. Kitchen appliances can be a danger to the infirmed individual as well as others, and must be looked at accordingly. Stoves, coffeepots, countertop ovens and toasters all can be dangerous if used in a neglectful fashion. Many home fires have been started with these seemingly benign household items.

Proper visual and hearing aids are essential to our comfort, safety, sociability and overall enjoyment of life. Provision of eyeglasses and hearing aids when necessary cannot be overlooked. Vanity may often overwhelm an aging individual's willingness to wear hearing aids, condemning those people to a world of silence, missed communications and ultimately exclusion from socializing with others. Encourage the use of such devices whenever the need arises, and assist the user in its proper maintenance. Failing batteries or ear wax plugging the ear piece may render the hearing aid non-functional. Seeing the appropriate eye or ear specialist on a periodic basis will help in this important area. An extra pair of eyeglasses should always be available.

When a family member has become disabled enough in some way that the operation of a motor vehicle creates a hazard to them and others, the family must intervene and remove the vehicle and make provisions for this person to have his or her mobility needs met. Here, one may encounter resistance and hostility from that person now losing his or her mobility independence. This is never an easy issue, but must be done lovingly and with alternatives. Whether this is accomplished by moving the family member into your home, providing an assisted living situation, Meals on Wheels, or daily visits and assistance from others in the family, intervention and problem solving must be addressed. The use of public transportation or taxicabs may also be appropriate, and each person may have different needs. If it is an issue of frank safety, appropriate intervention is a must. An automobile in incapable hands becomes a lethal weapon.

Nobody should be "voiceless." With longer life expectancy, we all must be cognizant that individuals all have varied and complex needs which they may not be able to articulate or handle themselves. Here is where friends and family become essential again. Seek the advice of the family physician and social services that are available in most communities. Again, sometimes trusted members of the clergy may be helpful and comforting to all concerned. Economic resources may be found in private insurance policies, Medicare and Medicaid funding or other local resources. Efforts made to plan ahead for these eventualities may result in a huge level of comfort for all concerned when their time of need arises.

Lastly, we must consider the importance of advanced directives from those now needing support and assistance from others. Most commonly, a document known as a "Living Will" and "Living Power of Attorney" can provide clear direction as to the individual's needs and wishes when they are no longer able to speak for themselves or when prolongation of life may be futile. The Living Will is a document usually prepared by an attorney with the express provisions made by the individual as to how they wish their end of life management to be handled. This refers to if and when the patient wishes emergency resuscitation efforts to be provided, under what circumstances they no longer wish for ongoing life support, how the individual wants his or her remains to be handled after death, etc. Clarifying these wishes before the need arises can go a long way to smoothing potential family conflicts, feelings of guilt, and providing a sense of empowerment and dignity to the individual or patient involved. The document known as the Living Power of Attorney further clarifies the wishes of the patient relative to financial and other personal needs, and who will be given these responsibilities when the patient can no longer act on their own behalf. Lastly, there is the Living Trust (Will) which is a legal document prepared by an attorney to stipulate the distribution of a person's assets after death. Planning ahead for these certainties can provide a great deal of comfort and clarity for all involved, and should be an essential part of everyone's planning. Information as well as certain documents can be found online for review. Again, having a qualified law professional help with these matters is essential. The copy of the Living Will should be made available to everyone involved in the patient's or loved ones care. Without it, the individuals express desires may not be carried out.

INSURANCE COMPANIES, MEDICARE, AND MEDICAID

We now arrive at the most bewildering, complex and variable component of contemporary healthcare, insurance. This topic has become so unbelievably complex, that one needs a degree in law, business administration and risk management to embrace it. Insurance companies, their policies, the actual insurance plans, and the current political winds seem to vary daily. It would appear that Congress itself does not clearly understand the full nature of the very legislation it has passed relative to healthcare reform. These issues are further muddled by complex lobbying efforts on the part of the insurance industry in conjunction with widely varying plans from region to region. I will make no effort to clarify these issues, as they remain nebulous to me and most others. I will, however, try to briefly distinguish between the basic differences and types of "coverage" available to us common folk.

Basically there exist five types of insurance. Of course an insurance professional may take issue with this breakdown, but here it is. Most of us have some form of this kind of health care coverage;

1) Indemnity Insurance
    a) traditionally reimbursed fee for service
    b) PPOs (preferred provider organizations)
2) Managed Care;
    a) HMOs (Health Maintenance Organizations)
    b) IPAs (independent practice associations)
3) Medicare
4) Medicaid
5) Champus/ Tricare (Military)

In order to better understand where we are today, again making reference to my "plumber" analogy in the introduction, let's look briefly how healthcare has been provided in the US over the last 50 years. For the sake of further simplification, I will reference Medicare separately, as it came about in 1965 during the Lyndon Johnson administration.

Traditionally, health care administration was a process between the doctor and the patient. The patient's health records and information were the private business of the patient and their doctor. Early on, you went to your doctor, or he or she came to you, and the doctor was simply paid a fee for his service much like today, when someone has his car repaired or house painted. In more rural areas, barter was commonplace. The "Doc" exchanged his services for those the patient could provide in return. For example, the country doctor may have delivered the farmer and wife's child in exchange for dairy products for a year.

Over time, there emerged an insurance product that would reimburse the patient for his healthcare costs, if the patient had such coverage, much in the way people are compensated by their property insurance carrier for casualty loss (property damage or loss). In the early 1980s we began to see the emergence of "managed care." Ostensibly the goal was to make healthcare coverage more widely available and less costly to the consumer.

Large insurance companies (e.g. Blue Cross, Aetna, etc.) decided to corral a vast number of medical consumers by going to the individuals and their businesses and offering healthcare insurance policies with lower premiums (cost). While capturing the majority of the market base, the insurance companies then went to the physicians, physician groups, and hospitals and said, "If you contract with our insurance company, we will provide a large patient base to you the health care providers." By accepting this contractual arrangement, the health care providers will accept insurance payment as payment in full, less a small patient co-pay, and at a big discount. We all quickly learned that when a large insurance company "owns" the patient market base, it is now in a very powerful position to control healthcare access, policy and costs, not to mention make a very large amount of money. The old adage, "He who controls the purse strings makes the rules," applies well here. No longer was care exclusively being delivered by the doctor or hospital to the patient, but there was a new player in this mix, the fiscal intermediary (insurance company). The patient now had a specified panel of "contracted providers" to select from and generally needed care preauthorization from the insurance company to get it. It was now a very different game.

Why didn't doctors do something to stop this abrupt and erosive change in health care delivery? The bottom line for physicians, particularly independent physicians, is that the insurance industry took powerful advantage through the old Sherman anti- trust laws which prevented non-contractually aligned physicians from getting together with other physicians and set fees for their services. Large legally bonded groups of physicians are better able to negotiate with the insurance companies. The independent physicians and small groups basically had to accept what the insurance companies chose to pay for their provider's services, because the insurance companies now controlled the majority of the paying patient base.

Physicians, who at one time may have received $500 for a service, were now receiving perhaps $125 for the same service, and usually months after the service was provided, if at all. One can only imagine the response to this by the medical community at large. The new bottom line today is this; we may often find ourselves with a lengthy wait to see a physician, and often not the one of our choosing. Visit times are now briefer and often less personal. Operating costs (overhead) for physicians have only increased over time and payment for services continues to decline. More and more physicians are moving toward elective cosmetic or fee for service encounters with patients and away from traditional health care delivery that will be managed by insurance companies. Those physicians that continue to actually provide traditional health care must see and treat far greater numbers of patients than they did in the past, just to meet expenses.

One can easily see how the degradation of our healthcare system will result in more system driven injuries and deaths. Medicine, in the traditional sense, has been profoundly disincentivized. Let's face it, nobody who has spent long years in training at great personal cost and sacrifice, wants to be told what his services are worth; if in fact the patient may receive these services; and if and when there will be payment to the provider of this care. Wrap all of this in a climate of inadequate to non-existent tort reform (legislation that regulates medical liability actions by attorneys), and you can better understand this explosive problem.

The bottom line is that things are not better. In fact, they have grown much worse. The existing supply of aging physicians, compared to the emerging demands of an aging and growing population, coupled with declining compensation for doctors, are having a profound effect on medical training enrollment. In many cases, this will produce challenges for the skill levels, training and quality of the providers themselves and will influence who will now choose to enter the field of medicine. This is a very alarming trend. I will leave it at that.

Now that you have a bit more insight into the forces that shape medical care today, let's examine very briefly the differences in the most common types of available plans.

Curiously, those that craft the legislation that regulates the insurance industry may hold themselves to different standards, and enjoy health care coverage unavailable to the rest of us.

Indemnity Insurance

Indemnity insurance is closest to the traditional forms of health insurance. Currently we will break it down to the more common types of insurance available to the consumer.

1) Basic Health Insurance: This type of insurance product says that the patient pays the insurance company a premium (insurance payment) and the insurance company reimburses the patient for his covered out of pocket health care expenses, usually minus a deductible percentage paid by the patient. If available, these plans can be quite costly, as the insured may seek care from whomever they choose.

2) PPO Plans: Preferred provider organizations are common plans, offered to individuals and by businesses to their employees as a benefit. The individual or business pays a certain monthly premium cost. That premium grants access to a panel of physicians, clinics and hospitals called Preferred Provider Organizations, which have agreed on a fee schedule and contracted with the insurance company. The patient (policy holder) usually has a deductible to meet and often a co-pay as well with each health care visit. This patient cost is intended to reduce frivolous medical care encounters on the part of the patient. Access to specialty care may or may not be regulated by the primary care doctor. Historically these plans had a lifetime maximum payment benefit. Payment for services or access to services remains at the discretion of the insurance company. Providers seen who are not within the contracted PPO network are considered "out of network" and are generally paid less than the in network provider, thus leaving you, the patient, with the obligation to pay the balance of the non-compensated fee. These plans may also not be "portable," meaning they may not transfer from one job to another if the insurance coverage was an employee benefit. All of the big insurance companies offer some variant of this type of plan.

Managed Care

This form of "Orwellian" care delivery, albeit socialistic, and concerning in content and methodology, is very commonplace as well. Let's try to simplify it and break it down for what it is. Objectivity is important here. Managed care is exactly that. Someone somewhere is managing your care and deciding if you shall receive it, from whom, and how much care will be allowed. We refer to this individual, who may be your family doctor, as the "gatekeeper." It is incumbent upon this gatekeeper to balance the care against cost. This conflict of interest potentially has a very dark side to it. I believe strongly that this conflict of interest flies directly in the face of the doctor's Hippocratic Oath. As a physician, to simultaneously be regulating care and its access based on cost, appears to me to be an unethical conflict. A caregiver cannot simultaneously deliver ethical, quality health care and be expected to ration it as well. Sadly, physicians have been placed in this very precarious position by the virtual monopolistic control the insurance industry now holds over private care access.

A large multi-specialty group of physicians with common management may offer HMO (Health Maintenance Organization) services, if that group chooses to practice within a managed care framework. Smaller independent groups of physicians who choose to offer managed care services to compete perhaps with larger groups, may choose to operate as an IPA (Independent Practice Association). Although the business bonds that bind the large and small groups together may vary, the model for care delivery is similar. The concept of Managed Care takes risk management and cost containment and places it in the hands of the medical providers (doctors) who deliver the service. This is a very disturbing turn of events when one carefully examines the conflicts involved.

Historically insurance companies have been paid by you the consumer to assume the bulk of the economic risk of your health care management, just as you have insurance against other casualty losses. The monthly or periodic amount paid to the insurance company on the consumer's behalf is called "premium." In the past, if you had insurance coverage, and became ill, the insurance company was obligated to pay your medical bills. Within this new IPA form of medical practice is where it gets very alarming. It is very important that the consumer understand the ethical conflicts and inherent dangers that may come with enrollment in a managed care program. The IPA, a relatively small group of otherwise non-economically connected doctors, get together and create this IPA. This IPA group of doctors now has the legal structure and ability to go to the insurance companies on behalf of this allied group of physicians and enter into a contract to assume the care for a large group of patients ("lives") who have purchased this form of health insurance. The insurance company turns over these patients to the IPA to manage all of their doctor-related care. The insurance company pays this contracting IPA a monthly lump sum based on a negotiated rate per member per month. This amount is called capitation. For example, the IPA may contract to care for a mix of patients of all ages and states of health, and the IPA may receive a capitation payment of $35 per member per month for primary care. It now becomes the responsibility of the IPA to manage the care of these patients regardless of how sick they are or how frequently they need to be seen by the doctor. Some patients will remain healthy and consume little or no care per month; some will require a great deal of care. It is now up to this IPA to regulate this. If the actual monthly IPA care costs provided are less than the amount paid by the insurance company to the IPA, the IPA makes money. If this capitated group of patients consumes a lot of care, the IPA makes no money and is on the hook for the uncompensated care. The bottom line is that the doctors in this IPA then don't get paid for the care they have rendered. The IPA is now placed in the position of "gate keeping" and rationing care. The doctors are now economically incentivized to give out less care than they are paid for, so they can make a living. What is also disturbing about this managed care concept is that the insurance company only pays a portion of what it collects from patient premium to the IPA. The insurance company ensures its own profitability by keeping some of this collected premium and passing the management risk on to the doctors! Remember, in the past, insurance companies were paid to take the "risk," not the doctors who are also delivering the care. IPA DOCTORS NOW MUST MANAGE THEIR MONTHLY CAPITATION PAYMENT FROM THE INSURANCE COMPANY. THE DOCTORS ARE NOW CONFLICTED BY THE NEED TO PROVIDE AND RATION PATIENT CARE. If the IPA provides "too much care," it fails to make a profit. This is absolutely nuts! Medical ethics and patient care go right out the window in many instances, yet this is now the basis for care delivery in many parts of our country. The only part of this mix with nothing to lose is the insurance company. Understand clearly, I am not telling you that quality is not available under this type of health care. I am cautioning you the consumer to be aware of this conflicted care model.

Let us now examine the HMO (Health Maintenance Organization). This model of healthcare is best characterized by a well-known organization that pioneered this concept many years ago in the San Francisco Bay area. This organization has grown very substantially throughout California and not only employs many physicians and ancillary health professionals within large multi-specialty clinics, but also operates its own hospitals. The medical staff are its employees. This entity has become the role model of the complete HMO. They seem to do it well. HMO insurance, like an IPA, usually carries a premium cost which is less than traditional indemnity or PPO insurance coverage. As an HMO patient, you will have a primary care provider (PCP) whom you must see or consult with prior to receiving any tests or specialty care within the HMO system. Your PCP is your" gatekeeper". Generally, without your PCP's referral you will not be seen by a specialist. In an HMO you often abdicate your ability to see the doctor of your choice. Often care in these environments moves along more slowly, as the referral process moves through the HMO system. There are "not for profit" HMOs and "for profit" HMOs. Generally both of these models must make money to remain in business. Profit can be made by withholding or denying care to the patient. For example, the primary care physician may choose to manage a problem best handled by a specialist referral. As with many insurance plans, as an HMO patient in the hospital, you will not likely remain in the hospital a minute longer than the HMO utilization staff allows. What your doctor thinks is appropriate may no longer hold much sway. Basically, you get what you pay for in life. If it is your desire to select your physicians and regulate your own care access, then a PPO plan is for you. If you are on a tight budget, or your employer only offers HMO type coverage, you must accept the risks and limitations applied by this kind of health care. Some HMOs are excellent in their scope of services, some are risky bare bones operations that I would use less flattering terms to describe. To further complicate the issue, there are insurance plans that are hybrids, mixtures of appealing and less appealing components that fit somewhere between a PPO and an HMO.

Keep in mind that selecting a health plan is a very major decision with significant potential consequences. IT IS UP TO YOU TO FULLY UNDERSTAND THE NATURE OF THE HEALTH INSURANCE PLAN YOU CHOOSE AND HOW THIS CHOICE WILL AFFECT YOUR CARE ACCESS AND PHYSICIAN SELECTION. If you are not clear on what you are receiving ASK QUESTIONS, speak with your friends, doctors, and your local medical society. Others may be helpful in your selection process. I cannot stress this enough.

MEDICARE AND MEDICAID

The last area to discuss will be the federally funded entity Medicare, and the state funded "safety net" called Medicaid. As you may know, both of these systems for health- care delivery are receiving a great deal of economic scrutiny, attempting to determine how they will fit into the future budget of our country, and their impact on the political fortunes of our rule makers. They both represent a huge public expense, and as of this writing may undergo significant future change. That being said, we can at least examine the system basics as of late 2011.

Medicare is a vast, federally funded entity which is broken down into several component parts. The majority of US citizens are eligible to receive Medicare coverage when they reach 65 years of age. There are exceptions to this, but they will not be discussed here. Medicare Part B is the patient benefit that provides for most physician related encounters. As a Medicare beneficiary, your doctor, assuming he or she is accepting Medicare patients in his or her practice, agrees to accept Medicare rates and payments for medical services, and generally electronically bills Medicare after the patient's visit. The patients have a co-pay for their care, generally 20% of the Medicare allowed cost of the service provided. In many instances, patients have a co-insurance policy (supplemental) that covers all or part of this 20% deductible expense. The doctor who treats Medicare patients is required by law to accept the Medicare fee schedule imposed as payment in full for his or her services. Medicare regularly publishes its fee schedule updates, so there is little mystery in how this works. Physicians, and other Medicare providers, submit charges with a CPT code for service in conjunction with an ICD-9 diagnosis code. Medicare then generally pays the doctor or provider 80% of the allowed fee and the patient, and or his supplemental insurance, pays the 20%

balance. A Medicare provider cannot charge any more or less than what Medicare allows for the service.

Hospital care generally involves Medicare Part A coverage. This only applies when your doctor admits you to the hospital as an inpatient. Part A applies as well to extended care coverage (nursing homes), home health care, and end of life care, generally referred to as Hospice Care. Deductibles are part of Part A coverage as well. Again, supplemental insurance coverage may represent a significant cost savings to the patient who has been hospitalized.

There are a number of different rules that apply depending on your age, how long you paid into the Social Security / Medicare System, if your spouse is eligible for Social Security, or if you are disabled. If you are uncertain as to your eligibility, then inquire through your Social Security Administration office or Medicare online (Medicare.gov). "Medicare and You," publication number CMS-10050 handbook, will describe your Medicare benefits and Medicare plan choices. You should automatically receive this publication upon Medicare enrollment.

Enrollment in Part A Medicare automatically makes you eligible for enrollment in Medicare Part B. You have a 7 month period in which to make up your mind about enrollment, or getting Part B coverage may become more expensive during the next open enrollment period the following year. Most people become eligible to begin the enrollment process 3 months prior to their 65th birthday. Whether you choose Part A or Part A and B, do not give up your existing health insurance before you have consulted with your insurance advisor and fully understand the implications of all of your options.

Medicare Part D coverage for prescription medications remains somewhat controversial, and is currently a work in progress. Your insurance advisor will be helpful in helping you understand how Part D may be of value to you.

Medicare Part C coverage relates to Medicare managed care through an HMO or PPO and has its own set of rules and requirements. Again, this component of Medicare will be best explained to you by your insurance advisor relative to cost and availability.

Medicaid is the state funded healthcare plan that generally provides "insurance coverage" for qualifying low income families and individuals who do not have, or cannot afford other forms of insurance coverage. Each state has a plan in force. Medicaid recipients generally have access to the same healthcare mechanisms as does an individual with private insurance and or Medicare. This is particularly true for hospitalizations. Physician care, particularly as an outpatient, requires seeing a doctor who will accept Medicaid patients, as Medicaid tends to pay physicians at a rate significantly below that of other insurers. Many physicians will see a certain number of Medicaid patients in their practices, not because it is economically remunerative, but because those physicians possess a strong sense of social conscience and a willingness to give back to their communities. Often, areas which contain large numbers of Medicaid recipients may have clinics which will provide for them and may be able to serve these patients in their native language, which is critical to effective communication. These clinics often offer a wide scope of additional out- patient services which may include perinatal care, pediatrics (specialty care for children), geriatrics (specialty care for older patients) and laboratory services to mention just a few. If you are a Medicaid recipient, you should be familiar with some of these clinics in your community. Medicaid funding is invariably a huge challenge to the budgets of our states, and now represents a fast growing socioeconomic problem. In light of declining reimbursement for all medical services, finding a physician within the private sector who will accept Medicaid patients is also growing more difficult. We must recognize that whether physicians or hospitals are compensated for their professional services, care is provided at a cost to the physician or hospital. This is broken down as a share of overhead costs, the costs businesses incur to keep their doors open. This cost of care provision is further driven by the attendant share of liability (medical malpractice insurance) costs borne by the providers (doctors and hospitals). All of these costs are going up, while the relative payment for services is declining. One can easily see that this has resulted in a growing care access problem.

The equitable distribution of healthcare throughout our nation will remain an ever-growing challenge. It is something that we all will need, and at some time, will necessitate making ourselves vulnerable to its intricacies and failings. Yes, we potentially have a terrific system, but it remains far from perfected. There remain special interests, political entities, and powerful lobbying forces which continue to shape medical care policy and drive costs. In part, greed, corruption and political influence have made our system of healthcare what it is today. We continue to struggle to provide care to all without meaningful tort reform. This places all of those medical providers (doctors and hospitals) at a tremendous disadvantage, insuring that costly, sometimes redundant, and often relatively needless care is prescribed. Constantly growing demands being placed on a relatively declining provider base create an environment where very dangerous errors can and will continue to occur. Inspite of a medical system with the best of intentions, there is no consistently available mechanism to protect all patients all of the time. No nation in history has been able to provide limitlessly for its people. The incalculable and sometimes misguided generosity of our country must eventually lead to systemic failure as we mandate provisions not only for ourselves, but for the people of other nations. As our medical care access issues degrade, it will lead to "dumbing down" of the whole system. After all, the road to hell is paved with good intentions. This simply means that if you do not look out for yourself or those you love, you must share in the responsibilities of less than perfect outcomes, or worse. PAY ATTENTION AND ADVOCATE FOR YOURSELF. Your survival may depend on it. Lastly, we challenge our medical and legislative leadership to begin to demand and to craft workable and effective methodologies in care improvement. Corporate greed and self-serving politics must be confronted for what they are. The priority should be the welfare of our people and those who provide for them. The fair and compassionate delivery of health care is one of the hallmarks of a great and civilized society. Somewhere along the line the lawmakers of the United States of America have decided that no people in this country, whether they reside here legally or not, shall go without state of the art health care, regardless of the patients' ability to pay for it. This legislation has placed enormous strain on what has proven to be a finite resource, and is clearly showing decline. There is nothing on the horizon which suggests that this profound social issue will be solved, or even improved. If we demand that a service is provided, then we must also make reasonable provisions to provide for and fund it. We cannot expect our best and brightest to flock to the altruistic career of medicine, knowing that they shall be conscripted into a crushing form of public servitude. Statistically, there is an ever-increasing risk of danger to the healthcare consumer. That is just the way it is! Until such time that there is a meaningful shift in this trend, we as consumers can only educate ourselves, advocate for ourselves, and beware.

THE AFFORDABLE CARE ACT "OBAMACARE"

This highly controversial piece of legislation was signed into law in March 2010. It represents governmental regulation of the administration and delivery of healthcare in the United States, and has profound and far-reaching implications on how we shall all receive care. It is now law. Whether it stands the test of time shall be determined. In light of the controversy that surrounds this legislation, access to care may further change in many ways. The key provisions of this piece of legislation are available online for anyone's review, and I would encourage you to at least read and understand the implications of these provisions on your particular healthcare needs. In light of many new insurance regulations, the Affordable Care Act is designed to "insure" an additional 32,000,000 people within the confines of the existing and relatively declining base of healthcare providers. Simply put, more patients, fewer doctors. This component of the legislation alone appears very much incompatible with the practical expectations of quality care delivery. It would appear that those actually tasked with providing the care had little, if anything to do with crafting this legislation. Such shortsightedness invariably results in unintended consequences for us all. Certainly one great truth remains. We cannot give to one, without taking from another.

One should draw their own conclusions about the impact and long term implications of this new law. We would also be well advised to carefully embrace the tenants of this booklet as we navigate through the future of US healthcare." Forewarned is forearmed."

WHAT IS ADVOCACY

Advocacy is simply defined as active support. When one advocates for another, one gets involved with the issues at hand. People advocate for themselves, or for others. Children depend on their parents to do this for them in many ways, and most of us will benefit at some time in our lives from the help or advocacy of others.

In a medical situation, advocacy takes the form of carefully listening to the input from the doctor or medical provider, asking appropriate questions when necessary, and on occasion, being the enabled "eyes and ears" for patients, particularly when they are unable or unwilling to do this for themselves. The previous chapters discussed these issues in some detail, and provide a good baseline from which to approach the issues of needed advocacy.

Hopefully with time, comprehensive patient care advocacy programs will emerge. They can assist patients in receiving the best possible care, and provide a" fire wall" for oversight and care related errors. When consumers better understand the value of medical advocacy, they will demand its availability. When our insurance industry understands the reduction in care-related errors and omissions, with improved outcomes, and greatly reduced costs, it too will demand and support such advocacy programs. When our care givers begin to embrace the obvious benefits of advocacy and oversight reduction, the natural tendency to react negatively to another skilled individual's oversight will be seen as supportive, and not threatening or intrusive.

We feel we have developed the framework for such a patient care advocacy program that we hope will stimulate productive thought and action, both on the part of our insurance industry and our lawmakers, but as well will be embraced by our overburdened system of health care delivery. Again, we believe such a system of advocacy will prove very effective at reducing care related injuries and deaths, and over time, significantly reduce the costs of quality care delivery.

We have the makings for the very best healthcare system in the world. This system must be fluid and reactive enough to embrace changes for the good of all involved. We sincerely hope you find this short booklet valuable and informative. Wishing you all the very best.

Respectfully,
Philip A. Scheinberg M.D., FACS
Linda A. Scheinberg R.N.

RESOURCES

Included is a listing of state Medical Licensing Boards and their respective contact information. These are only a few of the many resources available. Inquire whether there have been any significant disciplinary actions taken against your physician, or repetitive issues of professional malpractice. This information may be helpful in determining if your physician has the qualifications needed to provide the best possible care.

Most communities also have a local Medical Society, and most qualified physicians are participating members. These phone numbers should be available in your local phone book or online.

Check with your local hospital's medical staff office to be certain your doctor has hospital privileges, if in fact this is appropriate for his or her specialty.

Spend a bit of time doing your homework so you have the necessary assurances you are getting the best possible care. For personalized health insurance counseling and help making health coverage decisions contact;

State Health Insurance Assistance Program (SHIP); for your local SHIP phone number, visit

www.medicare.gov/contacts, or call 1-800-MEDICARE

MEDICAID: a joint Federal and state program that helps pay medical costs for some people with limited income and resources. www.medicare.gov, or call 1-800-MEDICARE.

SUPPLEMENTAL SECURITY INCOME (SSI); a monthly benefit paid by Social Security to people with limited income and resources who are disabled, blind, or 65 or older. www.socialsecurity.gov, or Social Security at 1-800-772-1213. TTY users should call 1-800-325-0778.

www.Healthgrades.com, Provides ratings and cost information for approximately 5000 hospitals and 16,000 nursing homes. Many Physician and Dentist profiles are also available through this site.

www.hrsa.gov, Provided by the US Dept. of Health and Human Services. Very informative site on multiple aspects of health-care delivery, care access, HIV/AIDS, maternal and child health, organ donation and transplantation, as well as many other aspects of Federally funded and supported programs.

MEDICARE;   www.medicare.gov
1-800-MEDICARE (1-800-633-4227

SOCIAL SECURITY;   www.socialsecurity.gov
1-800-772-1213

STATE MEDICAL LICENSING BOARDS;

Alabama State Board of Medical Examiners
PO Box 946
Montgomery, Al. 36101-0946   800-227-2606
www.albme.org

Alaska State Medical Board
550 W. Seventh Ave. Ste 1500
Anchorage, Ak. 99501-3567   907-269-8196
www.dced.state.ak.us/occ/pmed.htm

Arizona Medical Board
9545 E Doubletree Ranch Rd.
Scottsdale, Az. 85258-5539   877-255-2212
www.azmdboard.org

Arkansas State Medical Board
2100 Riverside Dr. Ste 220
Little Rock, Ar. 72202-1793   501-296-1802
www.armedicalboard.org

Medical Board of California
1426 Howe Ave. Ste. 54
Sacramento, Ca. 95825-3236   916-263-3100
www.ombc.ca.gov

Colorado Board of Medical Examiners
1560 Broadway Ste 1300
Denver, Co. 80202-5140   303-894-7690
www.dora.state.co.us/medical

Connecticut Medical Examining Board
PO Box 340308
Hartford, Ct. 06134-0308   860-509-7648
www.dph.state.ct.us

Delaware Board of Medical Practice
PO Box 1401
Dover, De. 19903   302-744-4507
www.professionallicensing.state.de.us

District of Columbia Board of Medicine
717 14th St. NW, Ste 600
Washington, D.C. 20010   202-724-4900
www.dchealth.dc.gov

Florida Board of Medicine Dept of Health
4052 Bald Cypress Way, BIN #C03
Tallahassee, Fla. 32399-3253   850-2454131
www.doh.state.fl.us

Georgia Composite State Board of Medical Examiners
2 Peachtree St. NW, 36th Floor
Atlanta, Ga. 30303-3465   404-656-3913
www.medicalboard.state.ga.us

Hawaii Board of Medical Examiners Dept of Commerce and
Consumer Affairs
PO Box 3469
Honolulu, Hi. 96813   808-586-3000
www.hawaii.gov/dcca/areas/pvl

Idaho State Board of Medicine

1755 Westgate Dr., Ste. 140
Boise, Id. 83720   208-327-7005
www.bom.state.id.us

Illinois Dept. of Financial and Professional Regulation
James R. Thompson Center
100 W. Randolph St., Ste 9-300
Chicago, Il. 60601   312-814-6910
www.idfpr.com

Indiana Professional Licensing Agency
402 W. Washington St., Room W072
Indianapolis, In. 46204   317-234-2060
www.in.gov/hpb

Iowa Board of Medical Examiners
400 S.W. Eighth St., Ste C
Des Moines, Ia. 50309-4686   515-281-5171
www.docboard.org/ia/ia_home.htm

Kansas Board of Healing Arts
235 SW Topeka Blvd.
Topeka, Ks 66603-3068   785-296-0852
www.ksbha.org

Kentucky Board of Medical Licensure
Hurstbourne Office Park
310 Whittington Pkwy., Ste 1B
Louisville, Ky. 40222-4916   502-429-7158
www.state.ky.us./agencies/kbml/

Louisiana State Board of Medical Examiners

630 Camp St.
New Orleans, La 70190-0250   504-568-6820
www.lsbme.org

Maine Board of Licensure in Medicine
137 State House Station
Augusta, Me 04333-0137   207-287-3601
www.docboard.org/me/me_home.htm

Maryland Board of Physicians
4201 Patterson Ave.
Baltimore, Md 21215-0095   410-764-4777
www.mbp.state.md.us

Massachusetts Board of Registration in Medicine
560 Harrison Ave., Ste. G-4
Boston, Mass 02118   617-654-9800
www.massmedboard.org

Michigan Bureau of Health Professions
PO Box 30670
Lansing, Mi 48909-8170   517-335-0918
www.michigan.gov/healthlicense

Minnesota Board of Medical Practice
University Park Plaza
2829 University Ave. SE, Ste 500
Minneapolis, Mn 55414-3246   612-617-2130
www.bmp.state.mn.us

Mississippi State Board of Medical Licensure
1867 Crane Ridge Dr, Ste 200B

Jackson, Ms 39216   601-987-3079
www.msbml.state.ms.us

Missouri State Board of Registration for the Healing Arts
3605 Missouri Blvd
PO Box 1335
Jefferson City, Mo 65102   573-751-3166
www.pr.mo.gov

Montana Board of Medical Examiners
PO Box 200513
Helena, Mt 59620-0513   406-841-2300
www.medicalboard.mt.gov

Nebraska Board of Medicine and Surgery
Health and Human Services
Regulation and Licensure
Credentialing Division
PO Box94986
Lincoln, Ne 68509-4986   402-471-2118
www.hhs.state.ne.us/reg/reg.index.htm

Nevada State Board of Medical Examiners
1105 Terminal Way, Ste 301
Reno, Nv 89502   775-6882559
www.medboard.nv.gov

New Hampshire Board of Medicine
2 Industrial Park Dr, Ste 8
Concord, NH 03301-8520   603-271-1203
www.nh.gov/medicine

New Jersey State Board of Medical Examiners
PO Box 183
Trenton, NJ 08625-0183   609-826-7100
www.state.nj.us/lps/ca/bme/bme.htm

New Mexico Medical Board
2055 So. Pacheco St, Bldg 400
Santa Fe, NM 87505   505-476-7220
www.stae.nm.us/nmbme

New York State Board for Medicine Licensure
State Board for Medicine, State Education Bldg., 2nd fl
89 Washington Ave
Albany, NY 12234   518-474-3817, ext. 560
www.op.nysed.gov

North Carolina Medical Board
PO Box 20007
Raleigh, NC 27619-0007   919-326-1100
www.ncmedboard.org

North Dakota State Board of Medical Examiners
City Center Plaza
418 E. Broadway Ave. Ste 12
Bismark, ND 58501   701-328-6500
www.mdbomex.com

State Medical Board of Ohio
77 So. High St., 17th fl
Columbus, Oh 43215-6127   614-466-3934
www.med.ohio.gov

Oklahoma State Board of Medical Licensure and Supervision
PO Box18256
Oklahoma City, Ok 73118-0256   405-848-6841
www.okmedicalboard.org

Oregon Board of Medical Examiners
1500 SW First Ave.
Portland, Or 97201-5826   503-229-5770
www.oregon.gov/

Pennsylvania State Board of Medicine
PO Box 2649
Harrisburg, Pa 17105-2649   717-783-1400
www.dos.state.pa.us

Rhode Island Board of Medical Licensure and Discipline
Dept of Health
Three Capitol Hill
Providence, RI 02908   401-222-2231
www.health.ri.gov/hsr/blmd

South Carolina Board of Medical Examiners
Dept of Labor, Licensing and Regulation
PO Box 11289
Columbia, SC 29211-1289   803-896-4500
www.llr.state.sc.us/pol/medical

Tennessee Board of Medical Examiners
425 Fifth Ave North, 1st Floor
Cordell Hull Bldg
Nashville, Tn 37247-1010   615-532-3202
www.2.state.tn.us/health/boards/me

Texas State Board of Medical Examiners
PO Box 2018
Austin, Tx 78768-2018   512-305-7010
www.tsbme.state.tx.us

Utah Dept of Commerce Division of Occupational and Professional Licensing
Physicians Licensing Board
PO Box 146741
Salt Lake City, Ut 84114   801-530-6628
www.dolp.utah.gov

Vermont Board of Medical Practice
PO Box 70
Burlington, Vt 05402-0070   802-657-4220
www.healthyvermonters.info//bmp//bmp.shtml

Virginia Board of Medicine
6603 West Broad St, 5th Floor
Richmond, Va 23230-1712   804-662-9900
www.dhp.state.va.us

Washington Medical Quality Assurance Commission
Dept of Health
PO Box 47865
Olympia, Wa 98504-7865   360-236-4700
https://fortress.wa.gov/doh/hpqa1/hps5/Medical/default.htm

West Virginia Board of Medicine
101 Dee Drive, Ste 103
Charlestown, WV 25311   304-558-2921
www.wvdhhr.org/wvbom

Wisconsin Medical Examining Board
Dept of Regulation and Licensing
PO Box 8935
Madison, Wi 53708-8935   608-266-2112
www.drl.state.wi.us

Wyoming Board of Medicine
211 West 19th St
Colony Bldg, 2nd Floor
Cheyenne, Wy 82002   800-438-5784
wyomedboard.state.wy.us

CPSIA information can be obtained at www.ICGtesting.com
Printed in the USA
LVOW01s1617061113

360255LV00017B/1036/P

[8]